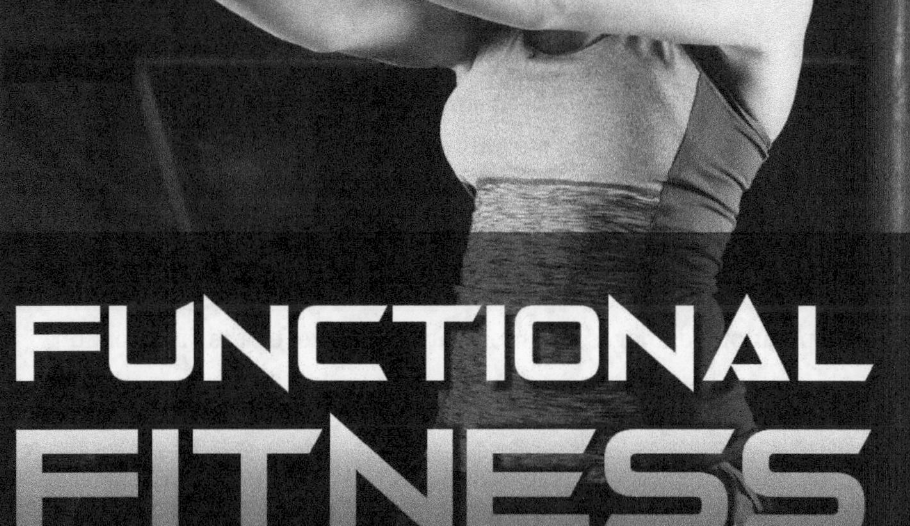

FUNCTIONAL FITNESS

Training Methodology For Real Life Application

the content within this book without the consent of the author or copyright owner. Legal action will be pursued if this is breached.

<u>Disclaimer Notice:</u>

Please note the information contained within this document is for educational and entertainment purposes only. Every attempt has been made to provide accurate, up to date and reliable complete information. No warranties of any kind are expressed or implied. Readers acknowledge that the author is not engaging in the rendering of legal, financial, medical or professional advice.

By reading this document, the reader agrees that under no circumstances are we responsible for any losses, direct or indirect, which are incurred as a result of the use of information contained within this document, including, but not limited to, —errors, omissions, or inaccuracies.

For Free Articles & Videos, Visit; www.lajaggard.com

TABLE OF CONTENTS

Introduction

When you say the word health, you are referring to the wellbeing of yourself or others. So naturally, health becomes a personal matter especially when it revolves around your own health. Everyone wants to be in better health which is again a very natural impulse.

The first and easiest things you can do to better your health is to eat properly and work out routinely. Eating properly can be dieting and monitoring what comes into your kitchen. Working out, on the other hand, can be somewhat trickier.

Working out doesn't mean you have to become a bodybuilder or weightlifter though those are possible achievements to gain from working out. It could simply mean you want to maintain a certain weight or keep your body moving properly and functionally. In such cases, to maintain proper health you don't need dumbbells and treadmills, only a functional fitness routine.

1

WHAT IS FUNCTIONAL FITNESS?

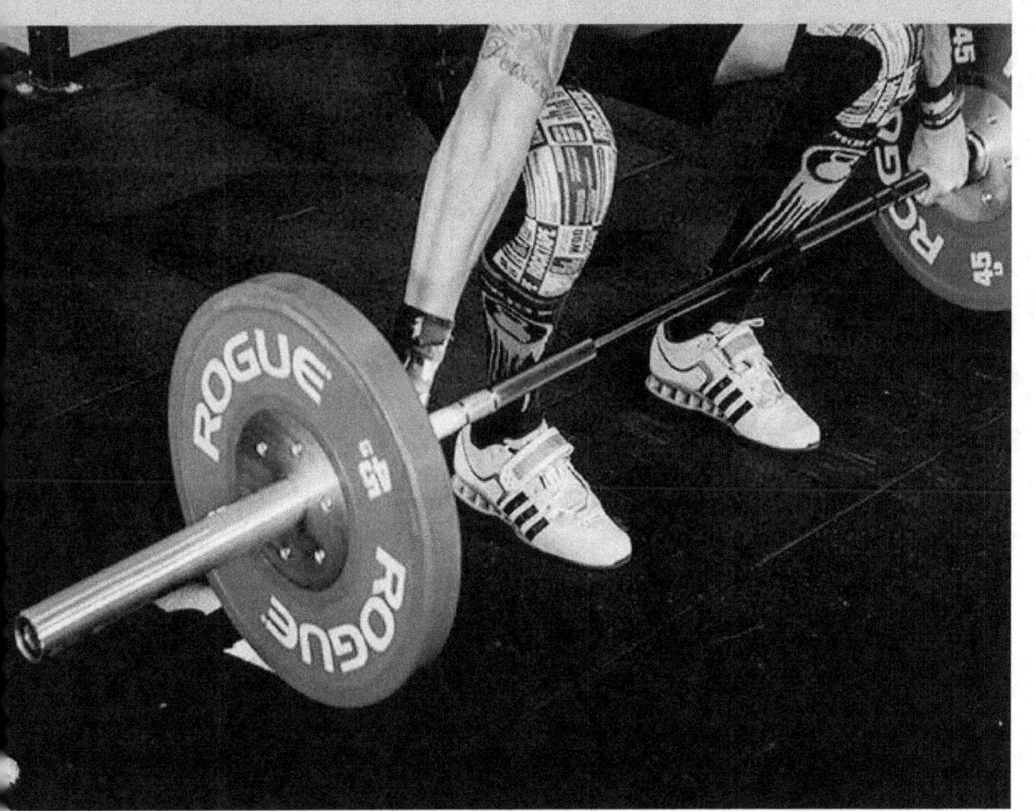

Chapter 1

What is Functional Fitness?

Functional Fitness Defined

You may not have heard of the term functional fitness before reading this, but the truth is that functional fitness is all around you. Functional fitness refers to a type of fitness where you keep your body moving in simulated routines that resemble everyday tasks.

Now, most people imagine working out as this fantastical imagery where you have a solid core and large protruding biceps that bulge every time you lift weights. This image is one that's better to burn. Not everyone can live this fantasy and in most cases, it's unrealistic and impractical. It's more difficult to maintain a bulky, muscular physique than a normal one, and not many people are aiming to become a PRO bodybuilder.

An easier and more reasonable way to maintain a fit figure is by sticking to simpler goals. What most people want is to be able to perform with the most practicality on a daily basis. To ensure this, drop the weights and stick to more natural movements. This is where you'll resort to functional fitness.

With functional fitness, you'll be doing squats, lunges, stretches, and pumps that are closer to home. All of these movements will resemble the actions you do in everyday life.

Take lunges as an example. Lunges are the movement of stretching out and bending your leg. Though you'll never be found walking in this cycle, it's imitating the movements you make in more extreme cases. Going up the stairs and running use the same actions as walking does, but with more strength and power. By doing lunges, your muscles and joints become accustomed to the strong pull and strain and therefore perform more effectively as you run.

As you grow older, you may have found that your body can't do the same things as it used to. It's alright since this happens to everybody. Unfortunately, the more lethargic you become, the faster this will happen to you. So it's better to get up and get moving in any way that you can.

Functional Fitness can be performed anywhere at any level of difficulties. For instance, you can even use your own body weight to perform the exercises without using any gym equipment. As long as you're moving in a way that can benefit your body, you're doing some kind of functional fitness. It's better than lifting the heaviest weights and then snapping when you're trying to load groceries into your car.

Complimenting Functional Fitness with Your Lifestyle

As mentioned earlier, hoping for the perfect 10 out of 10 body is unrealistic and quite impractical. The basic aim should always be maintaining a healthy body you as a person are satisfied with.

Being fit is only an extra benefit to yourself. That said, your exercises shouldn't interrupt your schedule, but rather flow inside of it. Once it becomes a problem to find time for your workout, a red flag should signal in your mind. Here are some tips to keep in mind when crafting a workout routine that works for you.

Firstly, it shouldn't take long at all. A 15 to 25-minute routine is enough to make a difference, so long as you're implementing this workout every day. You don't need anything that hard, just simple repetitive movements to properly pump your muscles. Your short workout can be early in the morning or after your busy day.

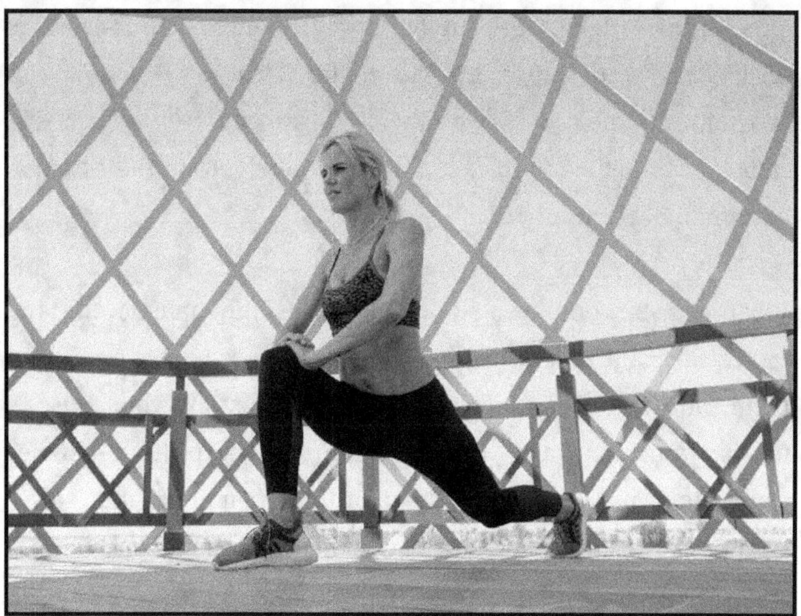

Typically, it's better to work out before you start your day's work, otherwise doing anything at the end of the day will tire you out more than you'd usually be. You can also develop intense strain and pain if you remain idle for too long after a workout.

Another idea is to spread out your workouts through the week. On days you're working, work out for only 15 minutes and on weekends or holidays, work out for 20-25 minutes. This way you won't tire yourself out when you have other things to do. Any system that suits your schedule is fine, so long as you're getting the essential minimum of 15 minutes.

When you start out, keep all of your moves minimalistic. Nothing too extravagant that'll pull your muscles before you've even used them. No weights in the beginning. They will strain your muscles far too quickly. Once you're used to the burn from simpler workouts, you can apply small two or three pound weights. Never start out big, as it's unhealthy, unrealistic and impractical.

When you're working out, keep some water nearby and put on your sports gear. Always keep yourself hydrated when working out and stay safe at all times.

Have lots of free space around you with a clean, carpeted floor or purchase yourself a yoga mat for moves where you bend or lie down. The more spacious your environment is, the safer it is to execute your workout effectively without injuring yourself.

Is Functional Fitness Right For You?

In contrast to popular belief, any given fitness program might not be a good fit for separate individuals. Though society has now made it something very normal, you may not fit in with this group of people that can work themselves to the bone.

If you're baffled, bear through for there is an explanation. Yes, it's true that functional fitness basically tries to cover all generic movements, reinforce your stamina, strength, and range of motion yet still, what about those people who can perform daily tasks and nothing more?

Illnesses, weakness, age, and injury can prevent you from doing more than what you're currently capable of. Though you may feel you're ready for more, your body may not be. Remember before anything else, there's no need to push limits that shouldn't be pushed.

In typical cases, functional fitness can cover most people's necessities. Whether you're hunting for a better body or a more productive day, functional fitness reaps the benefits to aid you down that road. But for those with physical restraints and disabilities, there's no harm in realizing what you're not capable of doing.

If you're injured, then it's momentary unless the after effect is lifelong. A scrape or bruise will put you down for a few days. Broken bones will keep you grounded for a much longer period and in some severe cases, the rest of your life. If bodily functions are really something you wish to improve though, then there's no reason for you to carelessly carry yourself around, injuring your limbs.

Other momentary obstacles can be surgery, pregnancy, traveling or moving and other impactful events in life. There's no way you can keep up working out each and every day especially if you have other things on your agenda to attend to. Fret not if you miss a day, simply get back into the routine as soon as you can. The longer you wait, the harder it'll be to return to your former glory.

As you grow older, you'll become more limited to what you can do. Bone health and newly developed issues have to be taken into account before you attempt any kind of workout.

Some people are born with permanent issues that prevent them from working in certain positions. There are many situations you may find yourself in; being born with weaker bone strength could mean you're incapable of working yourself past a certain degree. Breathing or digestive issues can also hold you down from working out since these areas will be directly affected.

CHAPTER 2

BENEFITS OF FUNCTIONAL FITNESS

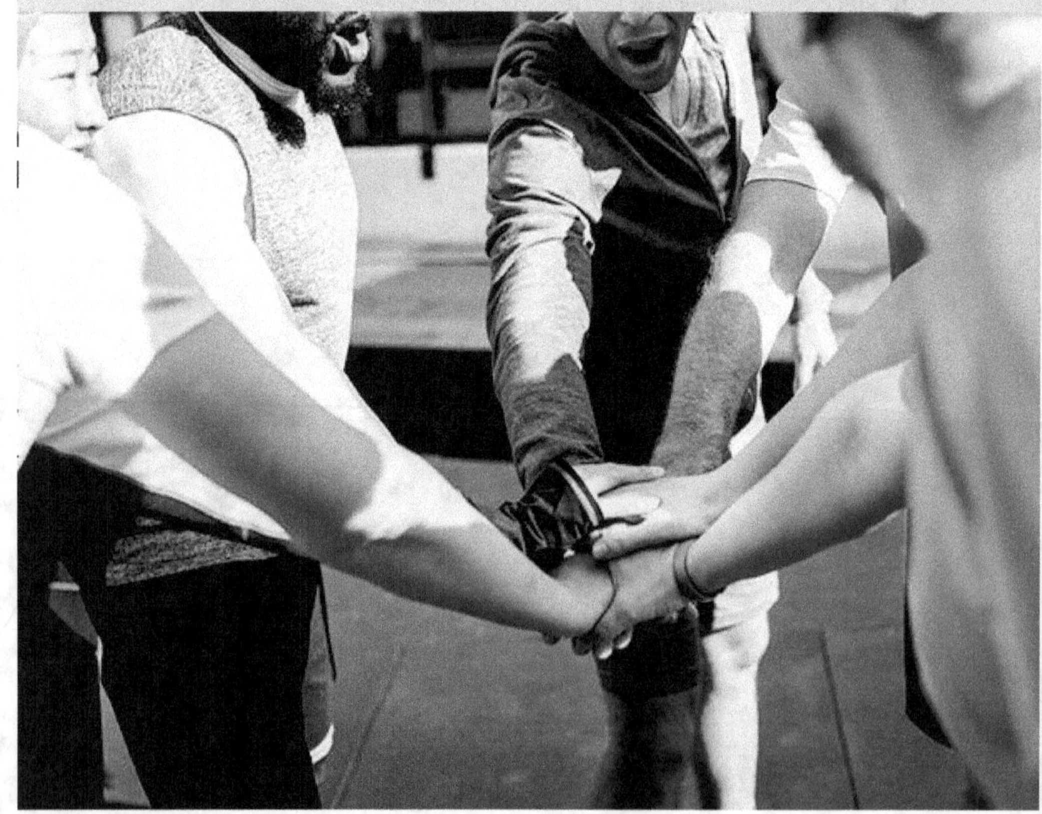

Chapter 2

Benefits of Functional Fitness

There are multiple benefits to functional fitness that can easily become part of your daily routine. To convince you further of the powerful impact functional fitness can have on your life, here are some benefits that functional fitness can provide you with.

Easier Movement

The more you practice, the better you will be in any exercise movement. Remember those days as an infant when you were clambering onto the furniture trying to figure out how to walk? Of course not, since you were after all an infant, but it's a perfect example for this point.

As an infant, you'd have always fallen over, cried a little, and then returned to your attempts to get up and walk. The more you did it, the better you got at doing it since your body steadily adjusted to the actions. The same procedure occurs when you're working out. The more you repeat these actions, the more accustomed your body gets to them and the easier they become to perform.

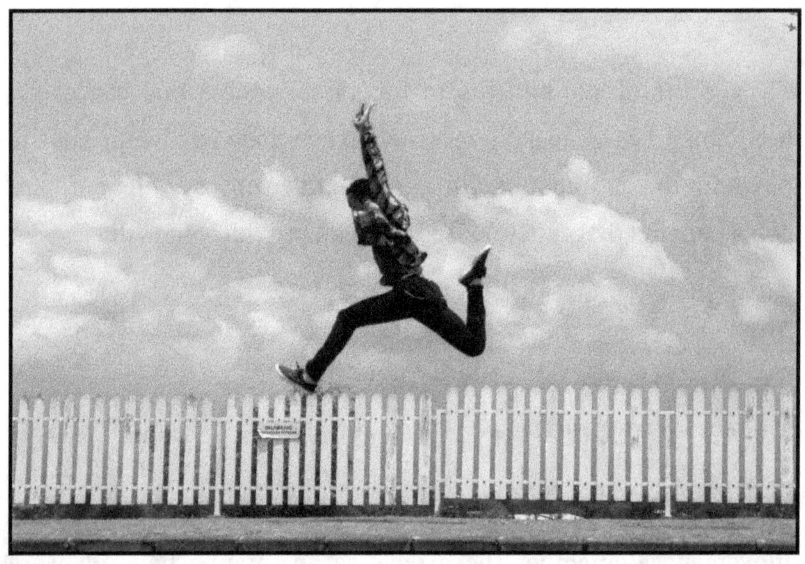

Once your body is used to these movements, running, bending down, jumping and heaving will all become a lot easier. That's why making functional fitness a daily part of your routine is so important. If you lose the momentum of working out regularly, you'll also lose the stability and consistency of your movements, and you may even get sore much quicker than you might have before.

The best part about functional fitness is that you can start anywhere with it. There's no grand expectation to meet or deadlines to pay up monthly subscription fees, just your own personal-made goals and free time.

Functional fitness in its most basic to most intense form will always remain a low impact workout. It means beginners can commence at an easy pace without the exhausting themselves. On the other hand, those who already have it implemented in their schedule will easily be able to pick up their pace without leaving their comfort zone.

Once you've gotten down the pattern of your functional fitness routine and you have a clear idea of what you're capable of, keeping yourself fit will never be easier. Movements are always done best in a flow. Without a system to your movements, you'll end up fumbling and tumbling in everything you do.

Practice makes perfect and this applies to everything. The more you do something, the more progress you'll endure to succumb to the best of your ability. So, for the best performance each day with fast and steady movements, functional fitness is the best solution to making your body perfectly functional.

Stronger Support and Immune System

Though you may not realize it immediately, when you work out your body becomes stronger. It's more resistant to attacks upon it. Now when saying attack, this doesn't refer to life threatening events, only simple accidents that can harm your body.

Scratches and bruises will have less effect on your body if you work out on the daily. Instead of having a throbbing bruise on your knee for days on end, it may hurt for a few hours and then feel like an irritating itch.

You'll also be able to handle more impact on your muscles while you're on the move. If running and going up the stairs were an issue before, working out can help you make those issues disappear. Functional fitness is the best kind of workout for improving your daily functional movements, since this is the primary focal point in all the exercises.

With each workout, you'll also feel a surge of adrenaline run through your veins, which is a good thing. Adrenaline gives you extra power and more stamina. When you need it, adrenaline will be provided to you at a faster rate than if you didn't work out.

Along with the buildup of adrenaline, there's also the buildup of stamina. With this, you'll be able to perform for longer periods of time and do more than you can usually do. If heaving the groceries tired you out before, then after proper functional fitness you'll be heaving more than bags with ease in no time.

Every day will be so much easier to conquer when your body is stronger and sturdier. You'll also feel more energized and confident as you grow stronger. Functional fitness can help you increase your general health in everyday life.

Functional fitness can also open more doors for you. You can try new sports or hobbies that involve going out with clearer certainty. With a newer, fitter you there is more you can do, more options you can discover. Stamina and strength aren't things you can develop overnight, but once you have them all of your days will change for the better. Walking to your work will seem less of a hassle. Running in the evening will appear to be more fun than irritating.

Though you'll never be able to compete with the heavy bodybuilders out there by only doing functional fitness, you can reach fuller potential in more material events in life. You can get a lot more done when you are functionally fit throughout your day.

Look Better, Feel Better

One thing everyone's been taught since youth is to always feel good about yourself. Though you may not dwell too much on this idea, it's actually a life changing mentality that can differentiate an optimist and a pessimist. Thinking positively about yourself is the key to a happier life for anyone's situation. Before accepting anyone else, accept yourself for who you are.

If you can't do that, then make yourself the person you want to be and accept that. If you feel negatively about yourself, it'll be hard to see anyone else positively. Negativity is an awful quality to have but unfortunately, it is more contagious than positivity.

So if you walk around with a hunched back and a grumpy expression all day, it's highly likely you're dampening someone else's morning even if that wasn't your intention. Rather than being the party pooper, try being the life of the party. Make yourself a more confident and happier person by working on the most important part of your life; yourself.

Functional fitness isn't that time demanding. All you need to do is honor 15 - 30 minutes of your time. Truth is, most people become self-conscious about their physique at some moment in their life. Maybe it had hit you in high school, your co-workers unintentionally made broad shoulders part of the uniform, or your in-laws pointed it out a little louder than they should've. In any case, the idea isn't to feel bad about yourself, but to feel motivated to do something about it.

With little pushes in the beginning, the results will start slipping into your jeans easier, show under your old sweaters and shirts and make your belts fall. Then, by that time you'll be able to work harder for stronger results that will truly dazzle your peers.

Though the steps to get there aren't small, they are possible and not hard to walk. Some great results from functional fitness are heightened strength in your joints and limbs, greater resistance against physical impacts and a better posture. That's right, with all the work you're inputting to your joints and limbs, your posture will be heavily impacted. A straighter back, a courageous lift underneath your chin and strong shoulders all come from 15 minutes of functional fitness every day. Isn't that something worth working for?

CHAPTER
3
FUNCTIONAL
FITNESS AND
OTHER EXERCISES

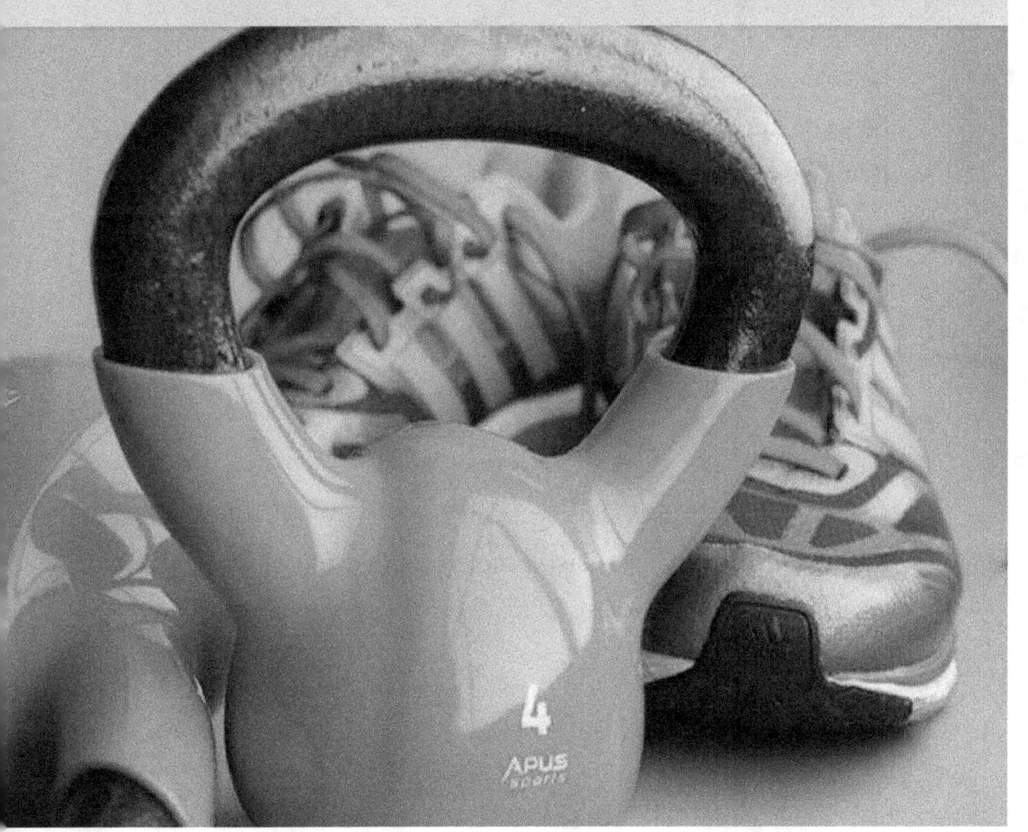

Chapter 3

Functional Fitness and Other Exercises

Functional fitness is commonly mistaken for any ordinary exercise and implemented into most typical workout sessions without anyone even realizing what it is. The fact is there's a difference between functional fitness and other exercises. Though the line between them may not be fully distinguishable at the moment, that'll all be cleared with the following comparisons between functional fitness and other types of exercises you may be familiar with.

1 - Bodybuilding

Bodybuilding focuses less on functional strength and overall mobility. Instead, it emphasize more on mind-muscle connection, time under tension for muscle synthesis. No doubt about it, bodybuilding-style programs are great for overall fitness, but it doesn't compliment all functional fitness has to offer.

There are similarities between the two types of workouts. They both do help make for a better, stronger, healthier physical appearance, though one exaggerates it more than the other. A fit appealing body is what you'll get, but when it comes to similarities, that's all there is. Sometimes you may find some functional fitness moves in your bodybuilding workout but you'll never find primarily bodybuilding moves in a functional fitness routine.

Functional fitness focuses less on grinding your muscles and more on your flexibility and higher standard strength in tasks you'll encounter. When it comes to the daily routine, functional fitness is the helping hand holding you steady while you work through the day.

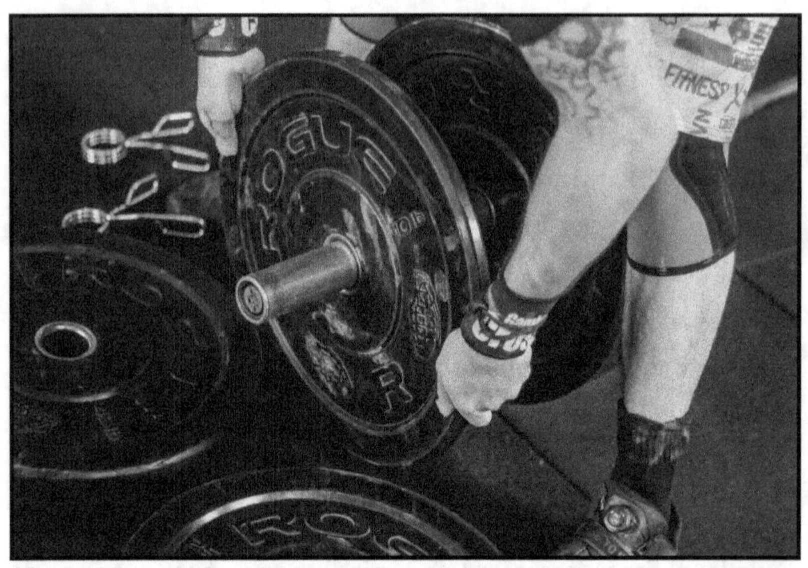

When you're a bodybuilder, being the handy average Joe isn't what you're aiming for. Instead, it's more like you're aiming to be the extraordinary model people look up to and gaze appreciatively towards. Bodybuilders are built to appear tough, but the truth is that they're not that tough.

When working on your muscles the bodybuilder way, the only thing you're doing is heightening the pulse and intensity of your muscles. Some core muscles in your limbs are completely skipped over and therefore not as strong as they could be. So while a bodybuilder has the look, they might not have the strength their muscles falsely portray.

Bodybuilders are actually pretty delicate. They can't take hardy impacts with swollen muscles and may have a harder time carrying themselves if they don't properly use their newfound power. When you're working out on a daily basis with the aim of greater performance in chores, you'll achieve that goal. When you work to make the perfect vision, then by all means you'll get what you want but then it's up to you to carry that proud physique.

2 - Heavy Weight Training

This is no stranger to most people's vocabulary. We've all seen how the strongmen in society lift the heaviest of weights with ease and blow our minds away. This is an extraordinary act indeed, but when will you ever do something that out of the ordinary in your daily life?

Functional fitness is quite similar to weightlifting and bodybuilding in various ways. You'll get the body and appearance you want and most likely more than those of a normal functional fitness routine. You'll also be able to lift amazingly heavy weights which is great, right? Not in every case.

In the gym it might be a bragging right, or when you're starting a conversation about your hard core hobbies. When it comes to working at home though, lifting a box off the floor might strain your back painfully, even if it's a light box.

As mentioned earlier, functional fitness works on your daily life, making tasks you do each day easier and less of a hassle to perform. Steadily, each chore becomes easier as you get better. Functional fitness figuratively lightens the weights on your shoulders that were placed there.

Weight lifters can easily lift weights off of their shoulders, but only when they are in the proper position, with enough strength and utilizing the right equipment. Those who weightlift obviously know that there are protocols and conditions to be met when becoming weightlifters. How to prop yourself with the equipment, how to hold the bar of the dumbbell, and how to keep posture when holding the weights airborne. These are all things you prepare to do when weightlifting.

An easier way to think of it is so; when becoming a weightlifter, you are preparing for the next meet, achieving the next Personal Best. When you're focusing on functional fitness, you're focusing more on preparing yourself for better health, mobility and the ability to handle daily activities with ease. So when it comes to practicality, functional fitness carries more weight.

Functional fitness targets if not all then most of the muscles you use on a daily basis. By gradually strengthening them through a series of exercises, they become more efficient and perform to higher degree. When weightlifting, you only focus on strengthening those muscles that will help you lift the heavy weights. This is fine as long as you are only planning on using those muscles for heavy lifting.

The primary issue when it comes to weightlifting is the way you're doing it. You're either propped in a seated position or lying down, a steady pose that isn't going to harm the rest of your body. After weightlifting for quite some time, weightlifters' muscles will become accustomed to this same pattern of movement in order to be more efficient with their lifts. However, when it comes to any other unconventional exercises out of their usual lifting patterns (such as Bench Press, Squats and Deadlifts), they often struggle.

3 - Group Training

When you're training by yourself in your own home, you have the luxury of comfort and solitude. Anything you're doing suits your needs. All you have to do is make an environment that's fit for fitness and you're well on your way towards a healthy lifestyle. The making of your new person is done by your hand, which is pressure on no one else but yourself.

What about when you work in a group? In a group you have an instructor, which is a hefty pro since they know what they're doing and teaching. When you're working with a professional instructor, there's a greater environment of motivation to endure the workouts for a better appearance and healthier body. Those people around you could be friends or at least acquaintances that want to achieve the same goal as you, making a friendly environment.

The environment itself is one carefully designed to cater the needs of a workout. So you have the proper space, the proper colleagues and the proper instructor. It sounds great so far.
Now here's where the hill drops. When you're working in a group, the catering isn't personal and generalized so that it fits a popular demand. Your demand may not be popular and you may find

difficulty keeping up with the crowd. If you have a disability or any type of illness that prevents you from performing certain actions, you may as well not be a part of the group.

When you're working by yourself the workout can be adapted to suit all of your own needs and run to your own pace rather than the pace of others and an instructor who is already fit as a fiddle. So keep in mind all the time what it is you're looking for from your workouts to decisively decide what it is you need and remember, functional fitness is a category of its own.

CHAPTER
4
COMMON MISTAKES
WITH FUNCTIONAL
FITNESS

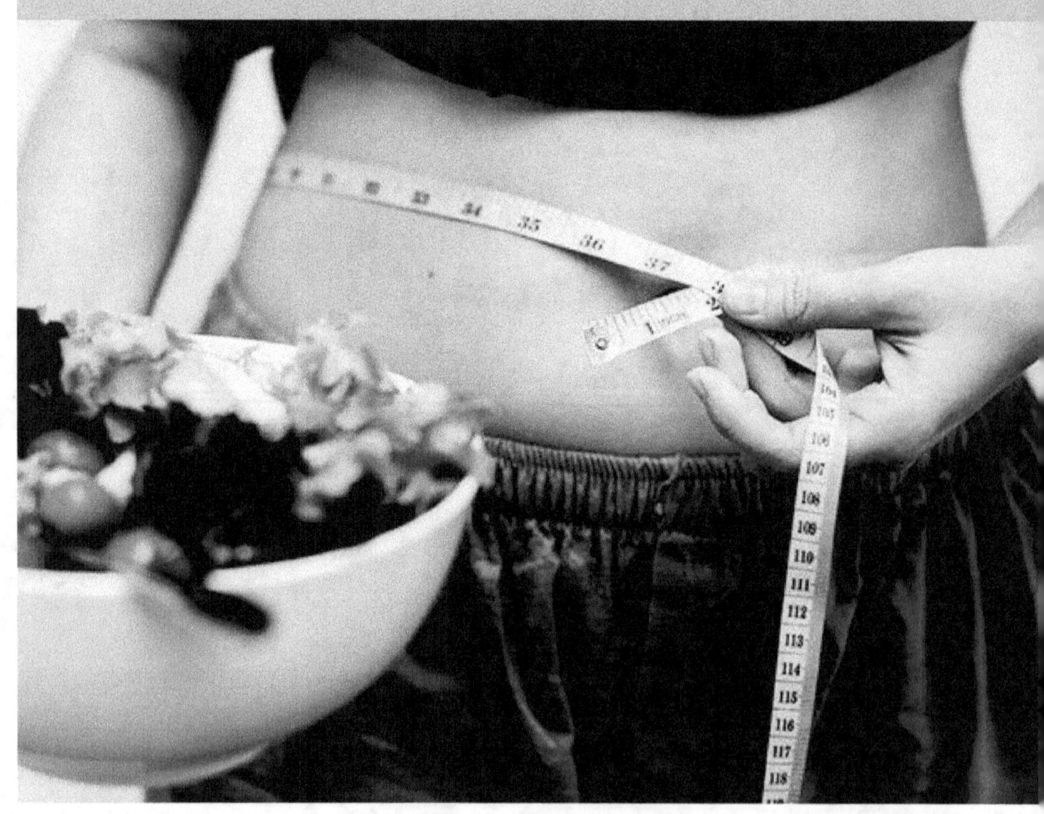

Chapter 4

Common Mistakes with Functional Fitness

Functional fitness is a great way to get yourself into shape, as long as you're doing it right. If you're confused, then the easiest way to word it is, you can work out wrong.

There are many common mistakes most people make when they start working out by themselves or even when they're starting out in a gym. So, before you start out on your own routine, make sure to do some research and learn the correct forms of execution.

An Everyday Routine

One mistake people tend to make all too often is doing the same workout every single day. If you do this, you'll never get the ideal muscles, tone, and body that you want. Yes, over time these workout sessions will get easier and you'll feel the strength in your limbs while doing this, but watch yourself crumble when you have to try a different workout.

Your body is made up of many limbs, muscles, bones and joints. If you don't work on all of these parts of your body equally, you'll end up with an imbalance in your strength and stamina which results in nothing good.

Any good workout will have multiple actions that'll target specific muscles in your body. When you combine the four main components of fitness (discussed in later chapters) you get the right balance between everything your body needs.

Unfortunately this isn't as easy as piecing a puzzle together. Instead, it's more like having to make smaller puzzles first in order to make a larger one. Once one component has been completed, you move on to the next one. This is a timely process which can't all be tackled in one workout.

So when one workout focuses on cardio and perhaps muscle building, another workout you do through the week can focus more on HIIT and stretching. Keep switching up your exercises rather than doing the same one each day. Take it slow, only change your routine when you know you can handle new moves and challenges.

If you constantly swap your daily exercise, you'll cover more ground quicker and spread the oncoming strength to all parts of your body. Only doing one type of exercise is going to tire you out and not properly help your body develop the way you'd have wanted it to.

Love What You Do

Some people work out because they feel they have to with no other choice. No one can truly determine your own situation quite like you can, but this is the wrong mentality. You should never approach your workout sessions with resentment. Always look to your workouts with optimism and confidence.

If you want to work out, then do it for yourself, not for anyone else's satisfaction. If you feel that you're being pressured into working out then the results are never going to satisfy you, even if you do make it to your goal.

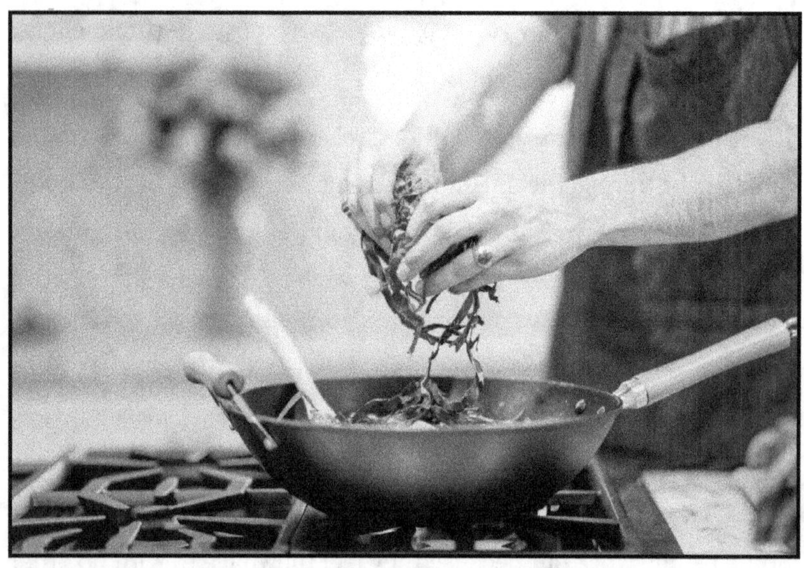

You have to enjoy something in order to achieve anything. If you don't like cooking, then you'll never enjoy a meal even if you mastered the recipe. The victory is always sweeter when you've got sugar, not salt.

Start working out when you feel good about working out. Do workouts that make you feel confident you have what it takes to make the change you need. If you don't like the criticism, comparisons or judgement of others, then don't go to the gym. You don't need to be in a crowd to get the motivation you need to starting lifting weights and running in evenings.

All your motivation should be positive, not negative. When you have positive motivation, it means you are being forward by the achievement you'll receive. When you have negative motivation, it means you are driven by the consequences of not acting. Don't be afraid of what people are going to say and do if you don't work out, think about all of the good response you'll get from doing so. Remember how happy you'll be when you finally reach where you want to be. Keep all of your thoughts positive and you'll not only feel good, but soon enough you'll look good as well.

Dieting

Another one of the most common mistakes people make when they're starting out, they think they have to start dieting! No matter what science and TV health programs try to tell you, dieting isn't the perfect solution for weight issues. Nowadays, people are coming to realize that diets actually limit you way too much.

When you start dieting, you work with either elimination or restriction. This should never be the case. Eat as much as you can permit yourself to. Have a balance of everything edible out there. Nothing should stop you from eating what you wish.

Just have a balance with what you eat. Most of your normal diet should consist of healthy hearty foods and whatever little snack your gluttony craves for can be satisfied once in a while. There is no issue with having a treat after some time. Keep control over how much junk food you have and keep that careful eye over your food to make sure the good always outweigh the bad.

Working out doesn't make dieting compulsory. If anything, it means you have to keep yourself energized more often. You'll crave more food once you start working out and that craving is one you're going to want to satisfy. If not, you'll become grumpy, hungry and your attitude towards working out won't be a very positive one.

Rolling with No Goals

There's no race to be won if there's no finish line. You always have to chart out your goals before you start working on a project.

In this case, the project is yourself, and you need to place some goals on what you want to do. Do you eventually want to have that hard core six pack? Are you aiming for a fitter, stronger you? Lay out your goal and make it clear to yourself, otherwise you may as well be running head first into fog.

Once believe you have a goal, set down your stepping stones to get there. You can't just hope you can make the jump from your side to the finish line. Make the bridge and cross it one tile at a time. It's a timely process, but it'll grant you the guaranteed success you want. It's better to work your way through at a decent pace rather than failing and having to restart the whole process.

First, try to lose weight. Aim for something that's fit and healthy. Go for at least 10 pounds less than what you are now. By the time you've reached that goal, you'll have gotten accustomed to the fatigue and strain after a hefty workout session. You'll also have a stronger understanding of how much you can handle and where the limit can't be breached.

Then, try aiming for another goal. Seek to tone your muscles a little bit at first, so you can understand how much time it takes you. Once you've gotten a clearer idea, you can start working hard to the final destination.

All of this will take a decent amount of time so don't give up if the results don't show after weeks, or maybe even a month. They'll come along soon and once they do it'll have been worth all of the time and effort.

CHAPTER
5
THE FIRST COMPONENT
OF FUNCTIONAL
FITNESS: POWER

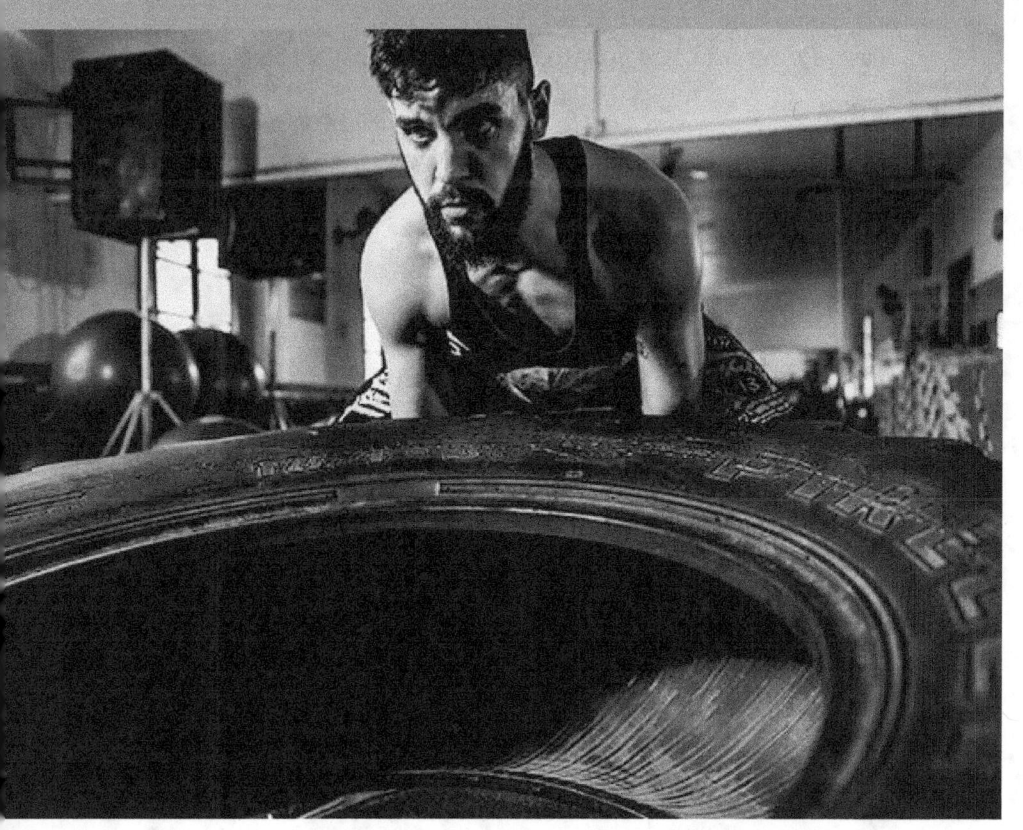

Chapter 5

The First Component of Functional Fitness: Power

When you first think of the word power, you may think of the word strength next. When it comes to working out though, this isn't the case. Power and strength are two different aspects when it comes to exercise, each targeting and influencing different parts of the body.

What is Power?

Power refers to your speed in doing something. When you're performing an act at high speed and fluency, such as jumping and running, this is referred to as your power.

Power does have other meaning in other situations, such as the power or influence you have over someone or a certain situation, but this does not apply to exercise.

When you say that somebody is powerful in terms of their physique, you refer to the speed it takes someone to do something. To clarify this point, consider the following example.

When you're capable of doing 50 push ups continuously, you're considered strong because of this capability. If you can do 50 push ups in two minutes, you'd be considered strong. But if the person next to you can do 50 push ups in half that time, they would be considered more powerful than you.

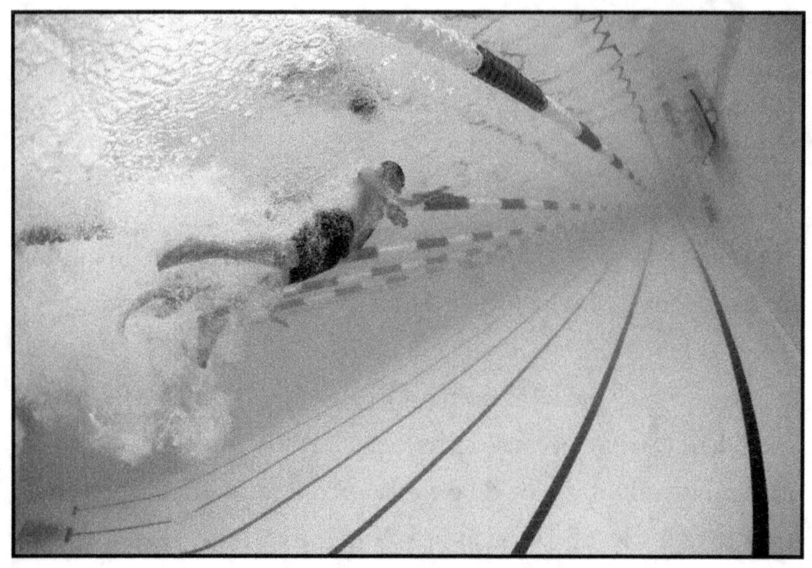

The same applies even when you're competing in sports. In swimming, if you and another person can only do 5 laps in one go, you're both as strong as each other. But if the person swimming alongside you can do it in seven minutes while you do it in ten, they're more powerful than you.

You can have the same level of strength as someone, but not the same level of power. Having the same amount of strength as someone isn't that hard to achieve as you may think. When it comes to having the same amount of power though, it becomes very challenging to find someone on the exact same level as you.

Don't get the wrong idea though, power and strength are both connected. Power actually is a combination of speed and the strength you have in order to do something. Without adequate strength, you won't have any power to exert.

You'll also find that over a period of time, you'll lose your power faster than you lose your strength. This is because overtime your body adjusts to wielding the strength it has, but as your body's original shape deteriorates over the years, your joints and muscles don't react as quickly as they would've done before.

Power is much harder to maintain than your level of power. The most common way to enhance your power would be by applying heavier weights to your workout so that you can perform your actions with greater resistance.

To further understand why you need to maintain your level of power, think of all the places where you need to be quicker and have more speed.

Power in your Daily Life

You can develop greater power to enhance your strength and speed. With all things you do, there's a certain amount of strength and ability required. Moving around items in your house requires strength you may not use on a daily basis. Cleaning for example, sweeping and dusting depend on a consistent movement of swaying your arm to and fro. You can have this strength to do to continuously, but do you have the power to do it quickly enough.

With power comes more valuable time in your grasp. How so? Think of all the things you have to do in one day. There are some things that will inevitably take time, like driving during traffic, waiting on the elevator and holding your spot in line during rush hour at the cafe. But during the day, there are things you can control such as climbing the stairs, walking or even getting ready in the morning.

If you can better the actions you have control over every day, you can spare yourself more time and energy for those things beyond your control. With more time you'll also have more stamina for the rest of your day. Some people are pooped after their daily morning routine and if that's you, then there's no way you're getting through the day on an energized positive principle.

You shouldn't be crawling on all fours to get through your day, you should be walking with stride each day, invigorated and prepared for the following days.

This is why you need power throughout your day. You don't have to be a strongman to have power. Any ordinary person can enhance their power to become a better more efficient version of themselves. Through progressive workouts you can improve your performance.

Think of power as the applications on a device to ease your understanding. Your phone would be your strength. With your phone you're able to call people anywhere you go. With applications, you can do more at faster speeds. You have access to social media and games. The more applications you have, the more you can do in less time. With only a phone, you have a base. With applications, you build up on that base to make it stronger.

Power Moves

A note to remember; when it comes to most exercise moves, they've already combined all four components of functional fitness into the exercise. The following exercises are examples of those that you can use to gain benefit in all fields including power, with these reasons further explained.

1. Jump squats

Jump squats are great for enhancing your core and leg power. This gives you the strength to withstand the resistance of squatting or simply bending down. With this move, you can bend your knees easier, knees being a primary area that wear out the fastest.

You don't have to jump in this move if it's your first time. You can simply squat to alleviate the strain off this motion.

2.   Dumbbell Curl

This move is by far the easiest to introduce to your workout. Take one dumbbell in each hand and curl your arms at a steady pace. This helps you improve your general arm strength.

With this, your arms won't succumb to heavy burdens when you pick up larger objects. The dumbbell curl can be made harder by holding your positions longer, introducing squats alongside the move or by lifting the dumbbells over your head and then dropping them before curling your arms. Of course all of these moves should be done after you're properly accustomed to regular dumbbell curves.

3.   Plyo Lateral Lunge

Rather than the usual lunge facing forward, take your lunges to the side. Stand straight with your arms down and move your left leg outward to the left. Stretch your left leg out so that it is straight, but your right leg is bent and go as far down as you comfortably can.

This will help your legs adapt to a side movement and strain from the upper body. This can help with extending your leg and bending down. When you feel comfortable with this move, introduce weights or resistance bands under your straightened leg. This will help the buildup strength in your legs.

4.   Burpee

This move is both as classic as it is functional. Your entire body's accustomed to general strain, from crouching to bending down to jumping all in one fluent move.

Start by going down with your knees bent to your chest and then pump them out so you're in a planking position. After doing this, bring your legs back to your chest and jump upwards. As soon as you land flat on your feet, repeat this cycle.

To make this slightly more challenging, bring your knees up to your chest while you're jumping. That way your jumps have a stronger spring to them.

6

THE SECOND COMPONENT OF FUNCTIONAL FITNESS: STRENGTH

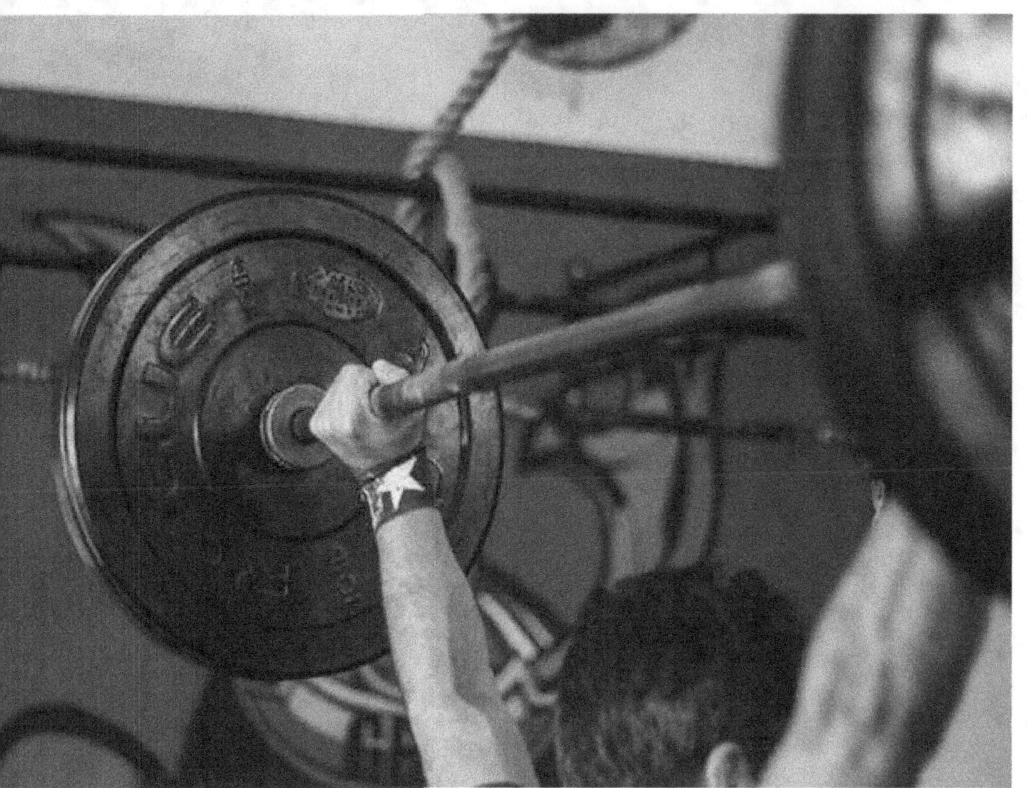

Chapter 6

The Second Component of Functional Fitness: Strength

Next on the list of components is the mighty force of strength. Strength is what most people tend to pay attention to, though it isn't the only thing that makes you a stronger person as a whole. Strength is the foundation you want to be sturdy and reliable in order for you to build over it.

What is Strength?

Strength has been mentioned in the previous chapter quite a bit, but never properly defined. Strength, when it comes to fitness, is defined as exerting force against some kind of resistance.

Everyone has their own level of strength; In your daily life, if you pay close attention to all you do, you'll come to realize that there are many times when you apply strength.

You'll also notice that not all strength is the same. There are different types of strength that you apply every day, those being;

1. **Maximum Strength.** This is the most amount of strength you can possibly exert in one go. Rolling your sleigh down the slide, you'll want to use your maximum strength to get the best push down for more fun. It's all you can do in the moment and if you have great strength levels, that's a lot of fun down the hillside.

2. **Elastic Strength.** This one needs slightly more explanation. Think of an elastic band and how fast it reacts when you let it go. It reacts similar to a whiplash, for a fast and extremely hardy impact. When you have elastic strength it means you're capable of reacting to resistance with a fast or elastic contraction.

3. **Strength Endurance.** This is the ability to repeat an action over and over at the same consistency. Think of a baseball player, mainly looking at the pitcher. Every time they throw the ball, they're expected to throw it at the same speed and force as the

last time they did before. This is where you'll note their strength endurance.

All these types of strength have their own focused exercises that help enhance your durability in these fields. Without these strengths, there'd be a lot you wouldn't be able to do. They can all also be specialized in. So if you only work on your strength and endurance, you may not have optimum elastic strength.

When it comes to all strength training, you focus on the muscles connected directly to your bones. These are the muscles that work directly with your movements and therefore have greater impact on how strong the outcome of your movement is.

Strength training is often the first item on any workout list since it's the foundation of all physical ability. When you have a sturdy enough base, you can move on to other focal exercises that centre other objectives to be dealt with.

If strength training isn't what you primarily targeted, then you may encounter issues with other workouts that turn out to be specialized in focusing on other functional aspects.

Strength in your Daily Life

You don't have to go to the gym to be strong.

Strength applies to all aspects of our life. You can be emotionally strong, mentally strong, socially strong and more. In this case, you're concentrating on your physical strength. Physical strength is used in every move you make. When you walk, run, jump, heave and shove, you're using your strength to do so.

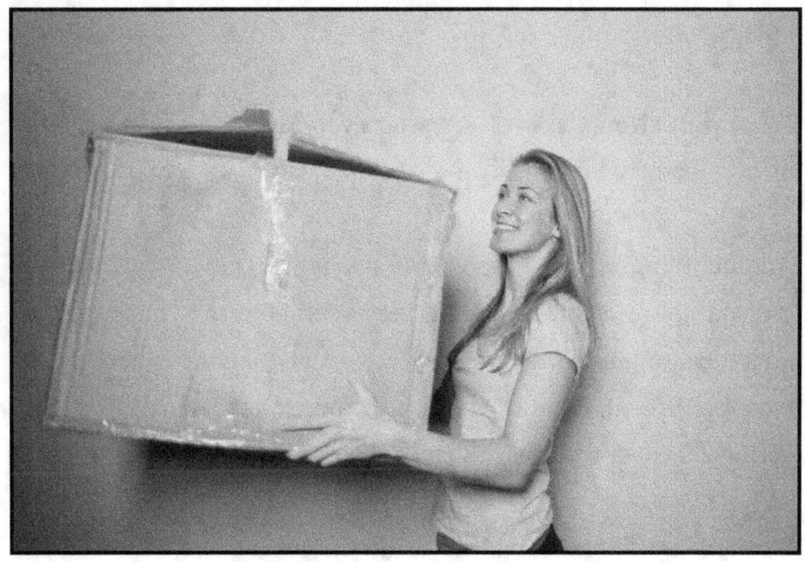

When heaving large boxes, you'll be using your maximum strength when picking one up. After that, it's maintenance of your strength level to carry the box to where it needs to be. If you do this action over and over again, you'll be using your strength endurance to withstand the constant strain created by the additional weights.

If for instance, the box slips from your hands while you're walking, you'd use your elastic strength to stabilize your grip. As soon as your box starts slipping, your reaction timing and elastic strength would work together to make sure you don't completely drop the box.

All of your strengths work together every day to make sure you're always ready to take the load of the day.

Another thing to note is that not all strength is trained with weights, but mainly resistance. Making the break between your exercises and repeating actions intensely are great ways to enhance your performance. Core workouts and complex sessions with greater variety all cover the muscles you need to bulk when working out.

Strength workouts should never be intense when you're starting out. They should be easy low level workouts with minimal variety. Your body needs to accustom to the new impact the workout is going to leave on you. You might have to take a break for the next 1 or 2 days if you're starting anew.

Strength Moves

Strength exercise should always target your entire body. Since strength has to be your foundation for all of your physical activities, it's better if you get all the body parts pumped and ready for action in one go.

Most exercise moves that emphasize strength will recommend the use of weights. So when it comes to creating a heavily strength exercise routine, weights, resistance bands and yoga balls are your key to finding the right way to truly test your limits.

1. Single Leg Bridge

In this move, you'll be coordinating your leg and core for dual coverage. Lying face up, lift your leg until it's at a 45 degrees into the air. Then lift your stomach a little to raise your leg higher. This move should be done as a pump, so that there's more burn with each repetition.

This move helps coordinate the core with the legs, resisting strain and pressure. You can implement this move with a crunch or with leg weights to make it more intense.

2.   Split Squat

With this squat, you make it harder for yourself, creating more strain and resistance. For this move you're not going to need weights, but a chair. Placing the chair behind you, place your foot on it so that one leg is bent and the other is straight. Then, step forward and squat with the leg not on the chair.

Do this with the other leg, swapping them to and fro until you feel the intense burn.

This means the workout is working and you're developing better leg strength.

3.   Glute Bridge

With this move, what you'll be doing is lying down on your back, and lifting your glute only in a pump movement. This will strengthen your core as a whole whenever you're going to bend or stretch your stomach.

You can place weights in your hands while lifting your stomach, lifting the weights to increase both your arm and core strength.

4.   Bent-Knee Calf Raise

For this workout you're going to need a box to step over. Stand straight on your box, arms straight down and legs spread shoulder width apart. Have a weight in each hand while they hang. Lift one of your legs up and have your other leg bent slightly on the box. Focus on concentric and eccentric movement of your calves while doing this for sets of 15-20 reps. Do this on each leg one after the other for greater effect.

CHAPTER

7

THE THIRD COMPONENT
OF FUNCTIONAL
FITNESS: RANGE OF MOTION

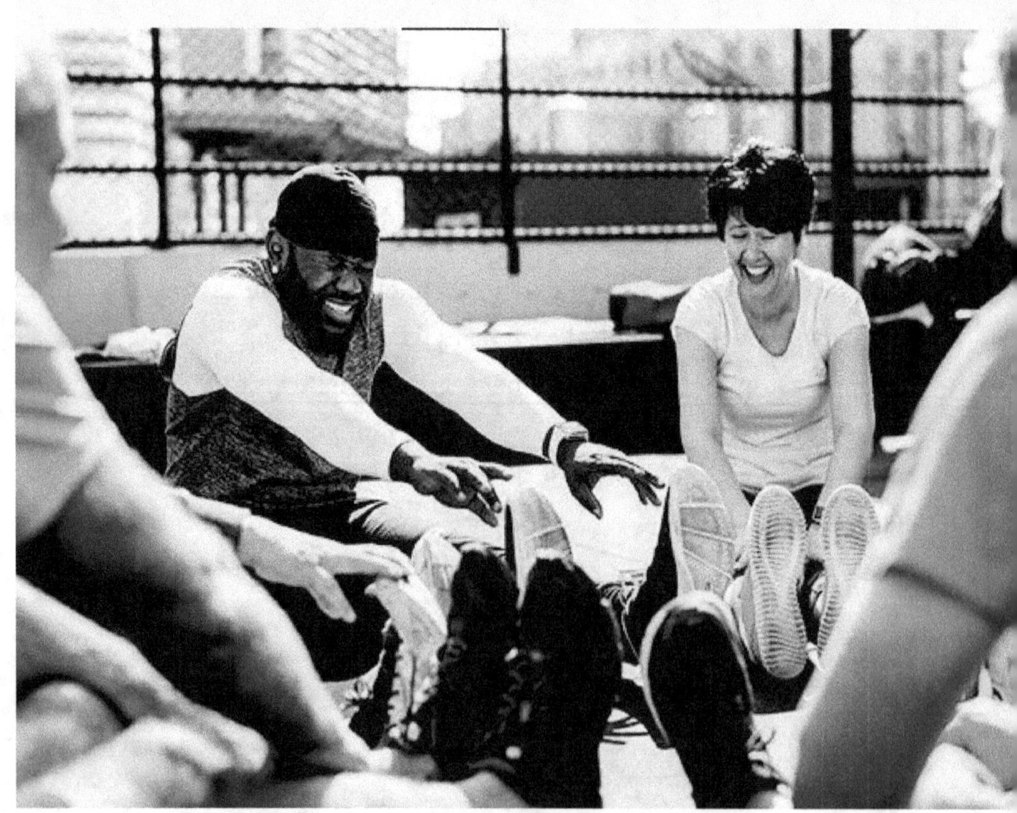

Chapter 7

The Third Component of Functional Fitness: Range of Motion

Next along the list of what contributes to your functional fitness workout is your range of motion. Your range of motion is defined as the measurement of movement around a specific body part.

What is Range of Motion?

Think of how far you can stretch your leg over the stairs. You might be able to stretch your leg to the second step, you might make it to the third. If you're tall enough, stretch all the way to the fourth but keep in mind, you're using your range of motion as you're doing this.

Range of motion can be associated with your flexibility, but they aren't entirely the same thing. Flexibility is the abstract movements your body can perform. Range of motion is quite literally the range of how far you can go. So, when you work on your flexibility, you're also working on extending your range of motion.

Your range of motion is what allows to extend your reach and keep your limbs alive, ready and always moving. Your range of motion relates to how well you can move around, how far your reach can go. Being strong is great, but if you can't reach the top shelf without stretching a muscle, then you're missing out on a few vital exercises.

Range of motion mainly comes from stretches. You should occasionally stretch your limbs in all directions where you can comfortably go. This way, you keep a hold of your range of motion. Range of motion is as easy to lose as your power is. Once you've lost the flow or routine of strengthening it, it's really hard to get it back.

Range of motion may not seem that important on its own but combined with the other components of functional fitness it really makes the difference between one person and another. You may have immense power and strength, but without a decisive range of motion, you'll never be the best runner since your legs aren't accustomed to taking such large steps.

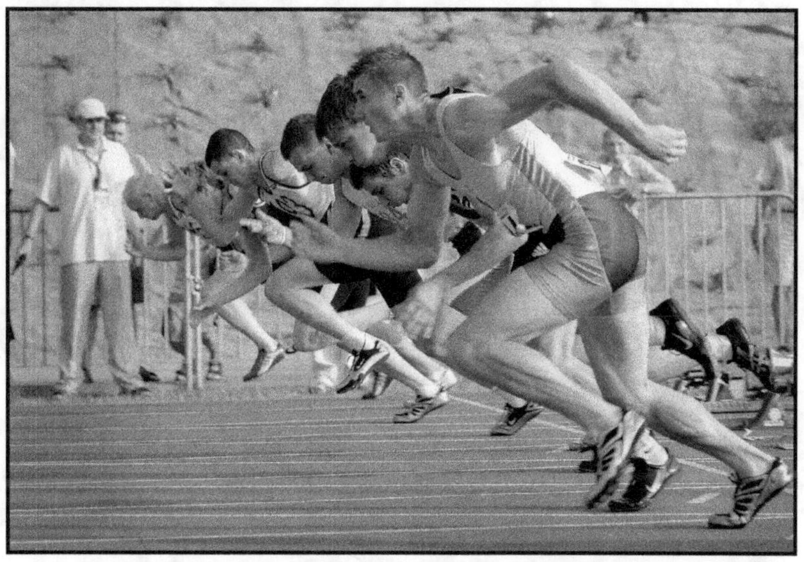

With power and strength, you can run consistently at a fast pace, which is good. To make yourself better, you'd improve the length of your stride by stretching your legs during exercises.

Never think of the components of functional fitness as isolation movements as they require multiple muscles synergy to perform each exercise. When they work together, they create a strong, sturdy base that you can rely on every single day.

Range of Motion in your Daily Life

Range of motion applies to everything you do, though you may not notice it in your daily actions. When you stretch to reach something overhead, when you take a longer stride to step over a puddle, when you kneel down to find something hidden under your bed, they're all examples of range of motion in your life.

When you work on your range of motion, you not only work on extending your reach, but also on making it easier for you to reach that far.

Think of the athletic performance that you can bring over to daily activities. It'll be easier to run, jump and walk at a faster pace. You can stretch overhead and below yourself effortlessly. Actions in general become much easier.

When you work out, you do actions in a more exaggerated manner than what they really are in real life. This technique ensures that anything you do in your daily routines remains something easily doable.

Range of motion isn't something you work on, on its own. It's interpreted with everything you do in real life and in your workout session. Though you'll find workouts that convey they are primarily range of motion workouts, they'll actually have a secondary focal point that additionally trains your range of motion.

The best part about training your range of motion is that it can be as easy as stretching in the morning. After you wake up, roll over to the side of the bed and stretch your arms over your head. Rattle your legs a little bit and arch your back. All of these can help day by day to make your reach a little better than it was yesterday.

Have a yoga session. Go out for a run. Doing the smallest of things can help your range of motion. The more you do it, the greater its development. So as long as you endlessly keep at it every day for even 15 minutes, you'll feel and see the difference.

Range of Motion Moves

These actions are better done in between at the beginning and in the end of your workout. All of these moves are done better when you hold them for minimum 20 seconds each.

1. Lunge with a Spinal Twist

It's the usual lunge with a new twist for you to try out. Once you're in the lunge stance, place one hand down on the floor and the other in the air, twisting your core so that you're facing upwards. Turn between your arms, taking your movements slowly.

This helps your core, leg and arm stretch. All is done in one move and the longer you hold it, the stronger the burn and the easier it'll be the next time you do it.

2.   Butterfly Stretch

Rather than stretching your limbs outwards, bring them all inwards so that you're comfortable in closed positions. Sit down and bring your feet together, making them touch each other's soles. Place your right hand on your left shin and left hand on right shin.

Keep this pose for as long as you can, standard 20 seconds to have best effect.

3.   Seated Shoulder Squeeze

In this move, you're sitting on the floor quite like how you did in the Butterfly Stretch, only this time you take your arms to your back and clasp them together. Immediately you should feel your shoulder bones constraining in the pose.

8

THE FOURTH COMPONENT OF FUNCTIONAL FITNESS: BALANCE AND ENDURANCE

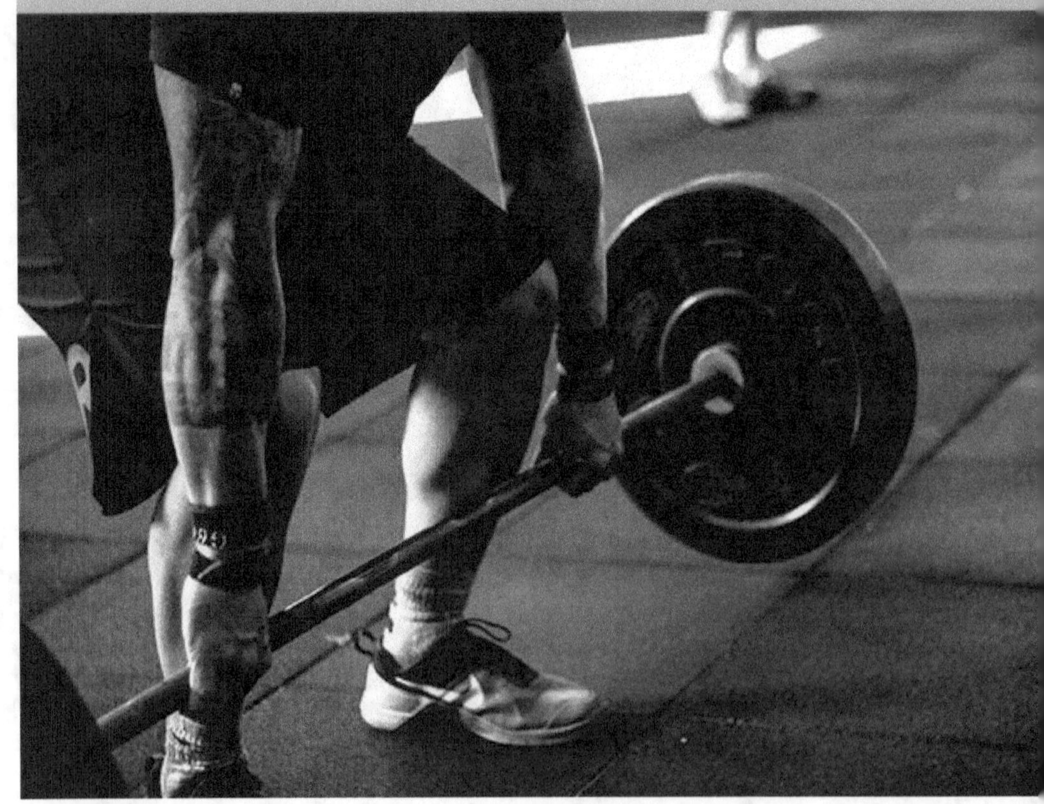

Chapter 8

The Fourth Component of Functional Fitness: Balance and Endurance

Finally, to complete the set of four, there's the last and final component, balance and endurance. These two work together in all ways and help enhance everything you can do, including the other components listed above.

What is Balance and Endurance?

Balance and endurance both have separate definitions. Balance is defined as your capability to control, handle and manage your body's movement. There are two types of balance to consider, those being your static balance and your dynamic balance. Static balance refers to the balance you must acquire while you're stagnant, completely still. This type of balance is easier to learn to control over your dynamic balance which is your level of balance when you're mobile.

An addition to balance would be coordination, which is a very important theory in fitness. Coordination is the capability to do two or more things at once, move your body in two or more different ways with fluency and efficiency.

Balance and coordination go hand in hand, and held in your other hand would be endurance. Endurance, which can also be referred to as stamina, is the ability of your muscles and body to remain active during a lengthy period of time.

Together, balance and endurance help create a set time limit of how long you can do something. With good balance and standard endurance, you'll be active for a long amount of time.

This leads to the final summary of all the components of functional fitness. With the proper amount of strength, you have a solid base to becoming a fit person. Your strength is going to help you withstand all the restraint you'll experience while you're working out.

Power is the speed that you can apply to your workouts to handle them quicker and with more force. Power helps build up your strength so that there's more to exert, helping you reach the extra mile.

The other way you're going to reach the extra mile is by using your range of motion, which is going to help reach further in a shorter amount of time. Don't get power and range of motion confused. Power will take you faster, range of motion will take you further. Together they create a useful duo.

Finally, there's your balance and endurance. They're the components that give you a time limit on how long you can last at peak performance. There's a limit to everything and eventually you'll wear down. Your balance will falter and your breaths harsher and raspier.

Put them all together and you have all of the pieces to create the perfect complete puzzle to understanding your maximized personal health.

Balance and Endurance in your Daily Life

Balance and endurance keep you running through the day in the most minimal way. They go together as well as rhymes do, harmoniously ensuring that you have the equity and stamina to progress through the events occurring all day. As the saying goes, everything works when there's a balance.

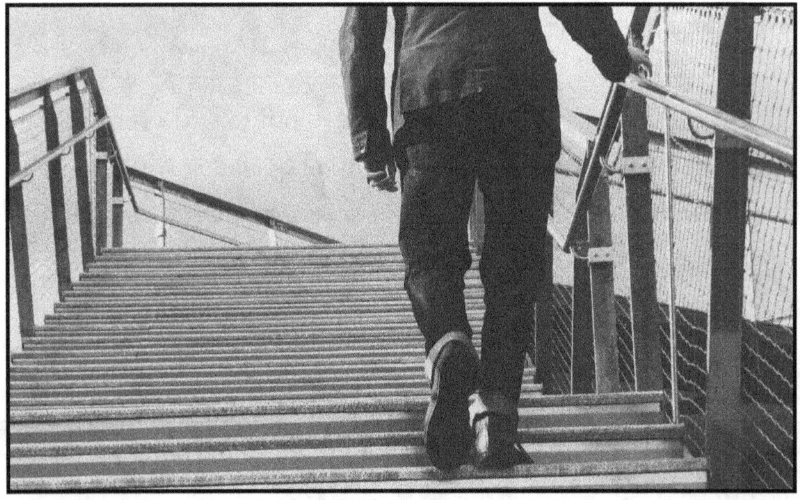

The simplest and most relatable example would have to be when going up the stairs. While going up the stairs, each moment you lift your foot is a split second of momentary balance. Without that balance, you'd go tumbling down the stairs.

In this case, you'd also require the stamina to keep going up flights of stairs. With the right amount of stamina, you can make it up the entire staircase, but without it you'll be wheezing after the third flight.

Balance and endurance are actually two things you can't notice quite easily. These two attributes keep improving on a daily basis, and contracting at the same time. The more you do in one day, the better you'll be tomorrow. The less you do today, the less you'll be able to do tomorrow.

If you consistently improve your balance and endurance, you'll consistently get better results. But balance, coordination and endurance aren't aspects you can simply stop working on. As soon as you find yourself on a suitable level of endurance, you keep at it.

Maintain your level and never fall from it. As you get older, it'll be harder to keep one level so it's better to maintain rather than trying to climb any higher. Just as well, if you stop working on them, your balance and endurance are going to fall by the day.

Cleaning, cooking, walking, talking these are all things that take up your endurance. Running, heaving, any sort of movement with any part of your body all require some balancing effort.

Without proper care, walking will become a chore and you'll become lethargic without the right level of stamina.

Balance and Endurance Moves

You can have a full yoga session once or twice a week to cover this type of workout.

1. One Leg Stand

With this workout, you'll be standing with one leg airborne and the other one rooted to the floor. Try holding this pose for as long as you can.

At first you might want to hold on to a wall or chair so you can better adjust to the pose. If your balance is generally not good, then start with your arms stretched outwards for greater balance.

If you have better balance, then complicate this easy step by pumping your elevated leg. This way you can better both your balance and your power with one move.

2.   Plyo Lunge

In this version of a lunge, every time you bend down over one leg, you're going to jump and swap to the other leg. In this manner you're going to help enhance your endurance with each swap, imitating the actions you do when running.

Plyo lunge is a more intense move than a normal lunge so please don't try it unless you're comfortable and more than capable of doing a regular lunge first.

3.   Straight-leg Calf Raise

With this move, your balance will be intensely tested. Standing on a step or box with your heels hanging over the edge, lift one leg behind yourself. Push your foot up so that you're on your toes, hold for a few seconds and then come back down. Swap your legs after a few pumps on each foot.

This is going to hurt when you do it, but you'll surely have better balance after this.

Conclusion

There's no perfect way to work out. Everyone has different needs and requirements, so there are different goals and ambitions that are always being followed.

Figure out what you want most out of any fitness program. Your goals can be easily achieved as long as you know your 'why' and dedicate yourself to it, so never falter your beliefs in yourself and take it the slow and simple way – Functional fitness will help you do just that. With all of the effort you put into yourself, the right amount of balance in everything you do and the courage to step up no matter what happens, you'll surely get what you need in the end.

To run, you have to first learn how to walk. To stop, you must first get started. For optimal health and functionality, functional fitness is the answer you've been looking for.

Visit Our Fitness Website at: www.lajaggard.com

www.ingramcontent.com/pod-product-compliance
Lightning Source LLC
Chambersburg PA
CBHW061727250726

48657CB00002B/813